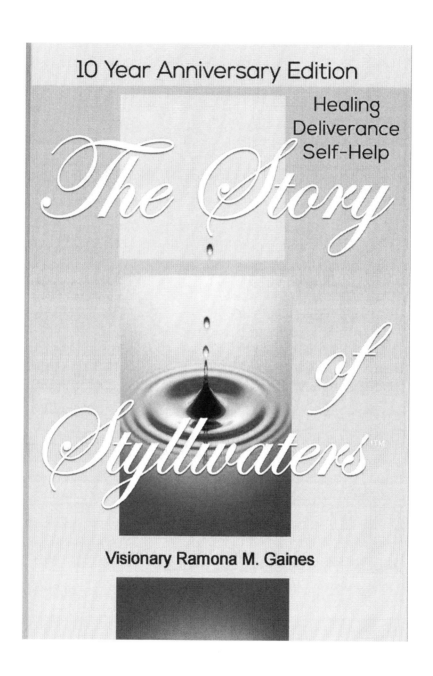

10 Year Anniversary Edition

Healing
Deliverance
Self-Help

The Story of Styllwaters™

Visionary Ramona M. Gaines

The Story of Styllwaters'

By Visionary Ramona M. Gaines

Published by Movement IS Medicine Publishing

www.visionaryramonamgaines.com

Cover Art and Design by Annette M. Carwell and Mashi Heshala

Dedication

First, I would like to thank God, my Daddy, for loving me and protecting me. Thank You for never letting me go, for watching over me from the cradle until now, for choosing me to be a vessel of honour even when I shunned and despised an honour that which I did not fully understand. Father, there is truly no one like You and I love You the more for it. You really truly are becoming, My Friend.

To my "Nanny" Ella Mae Gibson although you are gone in the physical you are still in my heart and the legacy that you left to me I will carry on with pride. I remember everyday that without God I would be nothing.

To my mother, "Big Rae Rae", you taught me so many lessons that I am just realizing. You taught how to paint my own picture if I did not like the one life gave me by sending me to art camp. You taught me how to dig up the weeds that I did not like growing around me and to plant my own flowers by teaching me how to garden. You taught me how to navigate through the waters of life by sending me to swim camp. I can doggie paddle, backstroke, breast stroke and wade through any storms because you taught me or made sure I learned how.

To my daughter Ellana Monae, my earthly treasure that is my gift from God. Thank you so much for your patience and understanding in all of our ups and downs. Remember, what I am doing now sets me free from my past and allows me to walk in the present and leave my legacy for you to carry on into the future

To Fantasia, because you made me believe again; Mary J. Blige for sharing your breakthrough experience and Jonathan Nelson and Purpose for letting me know that, "I Am Healed". My sister Prophetess Tracey Lynn Williams, thank you also for the push and your prayers to birth this again.

Table of Contents

Introduction

This story is the testimony of how God brought the Styllwaters' Ministry vision to pass, and what it took to get to this point of my jounery. It is not something that was an overnight process, however it has taken and is taking years of allowing God to process me and press out of me all that I have been through in order to use it for His glory. I have made many mistakes and fallen into many potholes, but all of what I went through was a part of my making. An important lesson that I have learned is to remember life is not supposed to make you bitter, it is

supposed to make you better.

Chapter 1

The Beginning of an Ending

On September 14, 1995, my grandmother Ella Mae Gibson passed and went home to be with the Lord. Up until that point I thought I had been living in Christ. You know, old things had passed away and behold all things had been made anew, so I thought. I really was at the beginig stages of knowing God and trusting Him like never before. I never really had a good relationship with my mother, so all that I had known as my mother was now gone with my grandmother passing. I know that the Bible says, "to be absent from the body is to be present with the Lord", and I was certain that my grandmother had gone on to be with the Lord. My spirit man could live with that, however, the little girl inside who still needed what she gave me was so lost, depressed and despondent.

My grandmother was stern but very loving to me. I spent most of my early childhood with her. When I became school age I spent holidays and summers with she and my grandfather at their home in Bristol, Pa. Bristol was a small quaint town just about thirty minutes outside of Philadelphia. Here were able to ride bikes, play kick ball, dodge ball and cathch lightening bugs most of the time. My grandmother or Nanny as I affectionately called her saw to it that some kind of childhood was preserved for me when I was in her care. She gave me stability, unconditional love and enough memories to last me a lifetime. They were memories of faith, family, food, and fun. But one of the greatest was my faith in Jesus Christ. I am convinced that I went straight from my mother's womb to church with my grandmother. She was very clear in her messages that without God she would be nothing. She often sang that song while cooking in the kitchen, "Without God I would be nothing, without God I would fail, without God, my life, my life would be nothing. I'd be like a ship without a sail". I grew to know and love this God one day for myself. I fell so deeply in love with Him. When I was seven years old I found myself at the front of Peniel Bapist Church with two other children my age accepting Jesus Christ as my Lord and Savior. One would think because we were so young we didn't understand what we were doing but I was very clear about what my actions meant and how I could not turn away because Jesus was drawing me closer to Him.

Prior to my Nanny passing away I battled with depression. Once she passed grief joined the party and became a daily part of my life. Now I guess you are wondering, "Well how old were you when your Nanny passed"? I was twenty-four years, but I was her baby and in that stage of life there is no one that could love me like my "Nanny", not even Jesus at that time. Now this many shock someone reading this but I must be brutally honest so you will know where I was and wehere God has brought me from. I knew that Jesus loved me and died for me and yes of course I did love Him. However, there was a place in my mind where I had placed my Nanny's love, even above the love of God.

I had exalted something or someone above the very God who blew the breath of life into my body and because of that and only that I became a living soul. Therefore, as you can see I had erected an altar in my mind that God had to bring down. Not that the very nature of the relationship was wrong, but it was my perspective of the relationship that was wrong.

In the book of Isaiah chapter 6 beginning of verse one, it says,

"In the year that King Uzziah died, I saw in a vision the Lord sitting on a throne, high and exalted, with the train of His royal robe filling the most holy part of the temple.

Isaiah 6:1 Amplified Bible

The is verse is exactly where I was at this point, a loved one had passed and God used this oportunity for me to see Him in the most Holy way and to enter in to the most holy place to have an intimate relationship with Him. No longer would I be an outer court dweller, but He was drawing me to the Holy of Holies so that I could be made new. In order for me to fulfill my destiny in Christ and to see Him high and lifted up as King and Kings and Lord of Lord the high place in my in my mind had to be brought down.

As you take this journey with me you will see the many times I tried to fill her void in my life. I felt like they would bring comfort and peace to my weary sould which was just longing for that place to call "home". According to Merriam Webster's one of the definitions of home is defined as,

"to the vital core".

I needed and longed for a social unit formed by a family (not necessarily your by societies standards) but a family was home to me. It wasn't a place but it was the way it felt to be in the presence that made me feel like "home". My Nanny was, "home" to me. Everything I believed that home was she captured the very essence of for me. After her death I kept trying to reinvent that core through different people (relationships), places (churches), and things (sex and alcohol). You might be reading this and saying to yourself, "How could church be a bad thing"? We, my answer is anything or place that exalts itself, or you higher than God is a high thing. church the building was never meant to replace a one-on-one relationship with God. Many times we run to the church wounded and expect it to be the thing that is going to fix all of our problems. The church is meant to be a guide, to point you to the ultimate One who can help you get your ship on course and stay on course. The reason we have so many wounded people in the church is because people have false expectations of the whole purpose of church. The primary goal of the church is to be a soul saving station. Once you are saved you are to be equipped for the work that God has called you to do, which we refer to as the perfecting of the saints for the work of the ministry. Then, once you have all that you need you are to go out to Jerusalem, Samaria and the uttermost parts of thw world. Depending on what your Jerusalem, Samaria, and uttermost are that is where you go. We all are assigned different territories and regions in the body of Christ and it is imperative that we make sure we are in our proper area in our right season. If not, we then run the risk of envy, jealousy, strife and so many other things that come about in the Body of Christ because of our disobedience by not following the will of God, or the pattern for our lives. Can we agree that God has already charted our course and that we are only walking out in the natural what has been done in the spirit.

Chapter 2

We Wear the Mask

I tried very hard to continue with life as usual once Nanny died. I tried to still uphold the traditions that she had instilled in me, and be the good girl she had told me to be. The key words here are, "I tried", and I failed oh so miserably because I tried to do it in my own strength. I never took that empty spot and allowed the Lord to fill the void that had been left. The thing was, my "Nanny's good girl" had a dark side and dark secrets that only she and I knew about and shared. Nanny never condoned what I did, she just never judged me. She loved me unconditionally no matter what. There was an unspeakable understanding between us that even spoke in the midst of the strongest silences. I had many things I always tried to keep neatly underneath the covers but I was only fooling the naked eye because God knew and so did those who had the gift of discernment. Months after the passing of my Grandmother, almost about two months I found out that I was seven months pregnant. Now I know you are saying there is no way in the world you could have walked around all that time and not have known you were pregnant, but it is the truth and I sure do not have any reason to lie at this point. I found out on November 10, 1995 when I went to see my doctor. I had a back injury due to a fall at work and had been in physical therapy for a couple months prior to this date. I requested that the doctor do an x-ray because after I would work the next morning when I went to get out of the bed I could not walk. I would have to crawl out of the bed to the hall closet and get a cane to pull myself up with it. I even had to begin to walk with the cane on a regular basis. Before the X-ray Technician took me back she asked me,"Was there a chance that I could be pregnant" and I said, "no". My doctor then said, "Once you are finished with the x-ray you can go home and I will call you with the results". I went in to get the x-ray done and before I knew it the x-ray technician was rushing me out of the room and told me to wait for the doctor. I immediately knew something was wrong so I said, "the doctor said I could go home and she would call me". She then said to me, "You have to wait and see the doctor before you go". So I waited and let me tell you that was the longest five minutes of my life. It almost felt like hours to me. In that short period of time, I had pronounced death, sickness and every disease over my young life. Anyone that knows me knows that my mind can go about a thousand miles a minute if you let it and man it was surely going. When the doctor finally called me in to the exam room she said, "Ms. Gaines we have discovered why your back has not healed, you are pregnant". I then said back to her, "If I am pregnant then I am very pregnant because I know the last time that I had sex". She then said back to me, "You are right, you are seven months pregnant, in your third trimester and could deliver any time now". The she put the x-ray up and I saw my baby fully developed in my belly. I felt like Sarah because at this point all of my friends had had their children and I assumed since I had never gotten pregnant, (not because I had not tried) that I was unable to have children. I then thought oh boy, I am not married, I am not with the father and I then I felt such sorrow because my grandmother would not be here to share in this with me. The doctor then told me of the risks of having the x-ray done and that they would have to do some othe testing to insure that they had not endangered the unborn fetus due to the radiactive wavelengths. She then congratulated me but I thought to myself thanks and oh by not so thanks because I was very unsure of what the road ahead of me was going to hold. The reality of this moment was that everyonewould know without a shadow of doubt that I was having sex. My reality was that I had been having sex for a very long time but was able to keep up the church girl façade when needed but had my private flings and affairs on the side. It was a yoke of bondage that I had gotten entangled in long ago and did not know how to get out it but honestly it was something that I loved. It was my way of releasing the stress and tension of my daily life. It was my escape drug, from dealing with the reality of life because in that moment I believed that person loved me and cared about me when in actuality they were only loving what they were getting from me and not the inner me that longed to be loved. I was constantly looking to fill a void that only God Himself could fill and would not sit still long enough to allow Him to do so. Like a junkie going thrugh withdrawal I was always searching for the next love jones, the next trip , tha next high. To be truthfully honest I was not loving any of them back either, I was using them just as well to get my selfish needs me and go on with my other life or the other person I needed to be for people. I always felt if I did the right thing I would be loved but if I did not I would not be loved. That is one of the true signs of a person that deals with the spirit of rejection. You will do anything to meet people's approval even live a lie and not be truthful to the real you. The real me needed help and deliverance, the real me needed to say I love Jesus but I hate myself. I hated what I saw when I looked in the mirror and now that the only person who ever loved me was gone I was feeling those feelings stronger than ever. Admitting that I needed help was so hard but because of the manifestation of the baby it drew attention to me in a light that was less than perfect and had brought my secret life to the forefront. What I had begun to look at as a bad thing turned out to actually be a good thing. I say that because a person can not get help until they identify the problem. It is not until you identify the problem that you can begin to come up with a solution. My problem was that I had a spirit of lust and I lived with the spirit of rejection and had eaten in its kitchen way too many times and even licked the pot clean. I did not love myself because if I had it would not have mattered who liked me or even loved me. My self-worth and self-esteem were shot; the need for me to be a people pleaser was birthed from my feelings of rejection and abandonment from my mother and my father. My mother was a hard and stern taskmaster, I would go as far to say that she was mean and wanted to break my spirit .

Our house was cold and dark and a place of solitary confinement for me. There wasn't any love there, any affection, hugs or kisses. My mother ruled our two-person household with an iron fist. The only thing I felt she responded to were my grades, which were almost perfect up until high school. I was the child who's parents made a xerox copy of their report cards and hung it on the refrigerator but never said, "good job" or "I am proud of you". Her behavior towards me reflected lack of care and nurturing. My Nanny on the other hand loved the very core of me inspite of me, whether I performed to her liking or not. I remember crying out to my mother telling her I felt ugly and didn't want to live anymore. My mother's response to me was, "Change your hairstyle or something". I remember writing my mother a note saying I didn't feel like she loved me and went to hug her and pushed me away. She was so hard and my heart was so tender and I needed so much but she was unable to give me what I needed. Then there were times when she would throw my feelings back in my face in front of company to belittle me for being soft. I was devasted that I could not trust my own mother with my private feelings and emotions. She was emotionally abusive when I ddn't get good grades, I could not get my hair done, I wasn't allowed to wear earrings or anything that would affirm me as a young lady. In some ways it was as if there was already a mold created for me to fit into and anytime I did anything different it upset the balance of nature.

Yet here I was about to be someone's mother. Becoming a parent scared me to death because I was convinced I wasn't going to do anything but screw up my unborn child's life. How could God trust me in this way because I just knew for sure I was going to fumble this play. This is what motivated me to at least begin the healing process of rebuilding and regrouping my life so tha I could have something to pass on as a legacy to my child whom I later found out was a baby girl.

So we began our new life together as mother and daughter; all the while during this process of us getting settled as a family I was still dealing with the effects of my grandmother's death. Our family was in the midst of great turmoil and it did not appear that it was going to get any better anytime soon. My grandfather was threatening to put me and my daughter out and eventually did.

So we left Bristol and moved in with a family friend in Philadelphia until I could get my head together. My daughter's father and his family were also a source of irritation to me during this time not to mention the strife and contention in church. Along with him deciding to not be sure whether he was or was not the father of our daughter. That was a little more than any one person could handle but I just kept praying through all of this and asking God to deliver me from my enemies and my foes. It wasn't that they were wrong about me, I had sinned, but no one choose to investigate the how's, when's of the why's. Truth is I had been sexually active since I was four years old. This is when my mother's boyfriend first molested me. When I was five years old in kindergarten my boyfriend Darryl and I had sex, (or what we thought was sex) in the teacher's bathroom at our daycare center. What I am trying to say here is that this problem is not something that just started but it had affected me from a very young age and there was no one to assist me with it or help me get delivered. My babysitter when I was seven years old had me watching soap operas everyday and taking in every seductive scene and envisioning myself in them. When I was nine years old I was having sex with a 14-year old boy and did not even understand that the semen running down my legs could have impregnated me if I had been menstruating. All I knew was that he was Rick and I was Monica of General Hospital and I was doing what I had I seen done so many times on television. We moved to another neighborhood when I was ten, it was a chance for a new start, new beginings and a new boyfriend. Do you see the patterns? It only took me a year and a half to begin to have sex with another boy in our new neighborhood. However this party got busted up early because his mom caught us and she didn't play that. My own mother found out and beat me almost to death. She put my head through a glass window, I thought she was going to kill me this day. By this time other things in my life had changed drastically, my mother became pregnant and gave birth to twins, a boy and a girl. Later on that year she got married to the father of the twins. The gentleman she married was not into me and she left me with and older couple in the neighborhood for them to babysit me while she, her husband and the twins would go and visit his family. This older couple had two grandsons living with them on the weekends and an older son that was mentally challenged. The son often would be in in his room mastrubating with his door open and as I walked up and down the stairs I would watch with great facination. Then one of the grandson's began to lure me upstairs to fool around. It gradually started off with petting and kissing. Then we began to have sex. I was twelve years old at this time. The older gentleman started getting wise to us because everytime the grandson would go upstairs so would I, until one day he told me to sit down and don't move. This did slow us down but it did not stop us. Each time I was just giving my body, my self-worth and self-esteem away. Eventually this behavior went into remission, I am not sure how and why but I know it did. For a while I went back to living as a child again. It was as if I slipped in and out of this lifestyle never ever being truly satisfied. All the while I was an "A" student and went to church every Sunday that I could, which was often.

By the time I got to high school I had slowed down a lot. I was more into sports and the school I went to was on the other side of town. There was no time for me to be hanging around the neighborhood and less trouble for me to get into. High school for me was not easy by any stretch of the imagination. The classes were hard and the teachers did not seem to understand me. They thought I was the lazy smart kid that could get it if I wanted to but I was not applying myself. The truth is that the school was very advanced and I was not prepared for this learning environment and their was no support system in place at home to help assist me in this transition. I knew how to study the answers but did not know how to problem solve and come up with the answers. M problem solving skills needed to be sharpened to say the least. As usual my mom was wrapped up in another man. By this time she had kicked her husband out there was so much drama behind that in our neighborhood that I had really been turned into hermit. I was not allowed to play, talk on the othe phone or have any interactions other than school or church functions with people my age and I was always babysitting the twins. I turned to God and basketball because they were the only things that brough me peace in my life. Nanny did not know the half of what was going on in my house but she would come and get me at least twice a month on the weekends and we would stay with her during the summer months.

I loved being with her and spending time with her. Nanny was my best friend. I believe that being with her in Bristol saved my life. I am grateful to have a place to escape and get away from what was a misreable life at home.

My mother never stopped dating and bringing men home to our house. But now she no longer allowed me to be apart of the family interactions. I guess having an older daughter was not so cute so I was treated like I was not apart of the family. My family along with my mother's boyfriends would all be in one room wathcing television together and I would be upstairs in my room alone. No television, radio and I was not even allowed to open my window for fresh air. I felt like I was a serving a life sentence that only seemed to be getting worse.

One night on the way home from basketball practice as I crossed the street after getting off the trolley. A car pulled up beside and it was a gentleman that had the exact resemblance of the man my mother was dating at the time. When he pulled up beside me he siad, "Your Mother sent me to pick you up", and because he looked like her friend I trusted him and before it was too late I was in the car. He still tried to keep up the pre-tense that my mom sent him to get me but I was not feeling right about this. So when we did not go straight to my house I kept asking when were we going to my house and he said, "In a minute". The he said, "We have to run and errand over the Gray's Ferry Bridge which I had no idea where it was. Before I knew it we were going over the Ben Franklin Bridge pulling up to a motel. He went inside, did something and came back out and said once I get to the room I could call my Mom. Immediately when I got into the room I picked up the phone to call my Mom and ther was no dial tone. He snatched the phone from me and threw me down on the bed and told me to shut-up and if I didn't he would punch me in my face. I thought this man was going to kill me. At this time in the news, so many young girls were being raped, killed and chopped up, I was convinced that I was going to be one of them. He ripped my underwear off of me and then forced himself inside of me. He told me my pussy was ready: he just kept repeating this over and over again. I faked like I was into it in hopes that this man would not kill me afterwards. I was so scared I thought that tonight was the night that I was going to die. So many thoughts raced through my head, "Where did my mother think I was", Would I ever see home again"? When he was done with me he told me to go get washed, and God knows I tried to wash it all out of me. I tried to pull it together so that he would trust that I would not tell and that I would make it home safely. When we went to leave the motel there was a wooded area on the other side of the parking lot and I just knew I was going to end up over there dead. To my surprise we both got back in the car and he drove back to Philadelphia. I vaguely told him in what vicinity to drop me off in so he would not know where I lived and walked home wondering what to do. Should I go home, would my my mother believe me? I went to my neighbors house where I went everyday after school and told her adult granddaughter what happened to me. The granddaughter took me home to tell my mother what happened. My worst fear came true my Mother did not believe me, she told me I was lying. The neighbor's granddaughter begged my mother to look at my face and to see I was not lying. The neighbor's granddaughter left and I was in the house with my mother who kept saying over and over again that I was lying. She said that I was pregnant and was trying to cover it up. She would not take me to the hospital, so my grandparents came down from Bristol called the police and took me to the hospital. When my grandmother go ther you could tell my mother had been talking to her and she was looking for holes in my story. My grandfather told them both to just get me to the hospital. The police sex crimes unit said for us to go to Jefferson Hospital that had a trauma unit for rape victims so we went there.

When I got to the intake unit of the hospital and the nurse was asking me questions my Mother kept saying, "I was lying". The nurse said to her, "You should be supporting your daughter". My mother's reply was, "Can I have some medication because I have a headache"? As I look back on that day and see my mother's face, I can see the pain of, "I can't belive this is happening", but at the time I did not feel that from her.

We were told to wait in the waiting room to be seen by a doctor. While waiting I was taken to take a pregnancy test which came back negative. So that dispelled all the thoughts that my mother had that I was trying to hide a pregnancy of an older man. I kept trying to sleep it away while waiting but my mother kept waking me up saing, "You're lying why won't you tell the truth". I kept saying, "I am not lying, I am not lying". I wanted to slap my mother to other side of the room. I just wanted her to let me sleep because I wanted more than anyone for this ugly nightmare to just go away. When I finally got into the room to be examined the doctor said that he could not tell whether I was raped or not. The police officer that happened to be a woman said that she did not believe me and said too that I was lying. She asked questions like, "Why didn't I jump out of the caror something, my answer is that fear had paralyzed me. Because I thought the man would try to kill me, they just did not understand the thoughts that were running through my mind. I was then given a pill by the doctor, which they now call the morning after pill in case of pregnancy and sent me home.

I was immediately sent to counseling which turned into family counseling and it was a disaster. I found no peace or solace there. I felt I had no voice so I just began to shutdown. I tried to forgive the man who raped me because that is what the Bible said but I hated my mother for not being there for me during this very dark period in my my life. I kept playing basketball and going to school but inside I was screaming help me please somebody help me!. Thoughts of suicide kept coming and going and I did try several times to end my life but nothing ever happened when I took the overdose of pills. I was still here living in hell with my mother, and to make matters worse she now wanted me tested for drugs because she claimed she did not undeerstand what was wrong with me, or why I was acting the way

I was. I hated her, life and myself in general. I kept crying out to God and by the spring of the following year I had re-dedicated my life to Christ and joined my grandparent's church in Bristol. God was the only thing that I could hold on to. I had accepted Christ as my Savior when was seven years old but then my Mother sent me to Catholic School and we started atteding Catholic Church. But for me there was something missing. I remember receiving my first Holy Communion and how when I walked down the aisle the song that was playing was, "Here I am Lord', and the very words of that song touched my soul. "Here I was Lord, I will go if you send and I will hold your people in my heart". Then the next year we received the sacrament of Confirmation, which they taught us meant that we would be endowed with power from the Holy Ghost. They had us dressed in red robes to signify the fire of the Holy Ghost but after the priest laid hands on me I felt absolutely nothing. I was looking for the day of Penetecost experience, the evidence of speaking in tongues fire and all. But I felt nothing. I had been praying hard and believing that God was going to show up in a very evident way in this service and it did not happen. Surely I thought in my mind after we had prayed all those rosary prayers, Hail Mary's, Our Father's that something would happen. The bible says to seek the Lord while he may be found call upon while He is near. I was calling oh yes I was, I was even yelling. When we said our prayers every morning in school I made sure I was the loudest one because I needed God to come see about me. I needed Him, but just could not seem to find Him the way I was looking until that Sunday morning, May 20, 1987. I felt Him and I found the Holy Ghost or should I say He found me. How do I know because I was sitting in the back of the church and do not remember how I made it to the front but I know I did and I know I felt the power of God like I knew I should all those other times. I know God was there all along but I needed to feel Him, to say I know He is real for me. I needed Him to be able to deal with my life and all of its ups and downs. I was dealing with so much hurt, and rejection and pain. My mother seemed to always be so angry and disappointed when she looked at me. I did not know where my father was but whatever had happened it had left my mother bitter and resentful and not able to deal with the reality of life and she was trying to fix the hurts of the past in her new marriage that failed and through my brother and sister. I loved my mother and hated her all at the same time. This was so confusing and complex, many in our neighborhood would try to intervene or help me through this place because they just did not understand why a woman would treat her own child this way. I have come to a conclusion; my Mother did not know what she was doing. She did not know the agony and pain she was causing me, all she knew was that she was a wounded little girl who never properly transitioned into life and found herself with a mini-version of herself much earlier than she expected and needed. The broke little girl became a broken woman that never had a chance to catch her breath and heal from her own life's hurts There were so many cracks in my heart that if I were a house in the hood I would have been infested with roaches and many families of mice. I was in bad need of repair. No matter whichever one happens there is still a breakdown. Many are walking around right now that have suffered breakdowns in some form or fashion right before your very eyes and you have no idea. They are people you deal within your everyday life; your hairdresser, your favourite Auntie that shops a lot, your co-worker that is on marriage number two, your boss or maybe even that mean nasty bus driver. Somewhere something broke in them one day and no one ever stopped to say, " Sis how can I help you in this broken place", or even give them the space and time do so. We just keep putting demand on top of demand on people and ourselves and then we look up and we have a bitter, nasty, mean-spirited woman looking at us in the mirror that we don't like and neither does anyone else.

Chapter 3

Selah

You know when I was in my senior year of high school my teacher asked us what we wanted out of life. Many said cars, houses, careers, fortune and fame. I said, "Peace of mind". The whole class and even my teacher thought that was a rather heavy statement for a seventeen year-old but to me I felt that it was essential in order to live your life to the fullest and to experience all that it had to offer. Even then I knew I was looking for whay I needed in the wrong people, places and thngs. There were so many cracks in my heart that if I were a house in the hood I would have been infested with roaches and many families of mice. I was in bad need of repair. But yet on the outside I looked so neathly packaged, I looked like I had it all together. I had gotten myself together academically so that I could get into college. This is what my mother and family had worked for and I was determined to deliver. One of the things I love my mother for is this; she saw to it that I got the best education I know I won't ever know all that she sacraficed for me to do o but I know that she did. Mom for that I will always be grateful.

In church I knew what to say and when to say it to have the right effect and to not tip anyone off that a lot of things were amiss. In my neighborhood I was the catholic schoolgirl who discreetly handled her business and many respected and admired me for that although I will never understand why. Not manh knew I hated my Mother and no longer repected her. I felt burdened with the responsibility of raising her two children who by the way I did not consent to being born eleven years after me. I decided to go to college not to get and education but to get away from the in-house babysitting job. If you were to see my college transcripts today you would see this was very evident. If you remember the song, "My Girl Loves to Party All the Time", well that was me in college. I was partying all the time but still seeking out God. Yes I was faithful in church and the works of church but was failing in my relationship with God because I still would not sit still for the healing that I knew I needed. I would invite God in but would not allow Him to what I asked Him to come in and do. It was like me paying a contractor to come in and remodel my home, he has all the materials there and then you say you don't have to start yet. Or better yet us telling him how to do his job and he is the expert. I am sure that there many times when God said, "Why did she even invite me in if she was not going to give me full control"? Like how many times have we all said, "Have your way to God and then went off and made our own decisions and still did our own thing? I can speak for myself and say I have done it way more times than I care to count.

Chapter 4

Labor Pains

When I received the vision for Styllwaters' Café, I was in the midst of the worst places in my lifeyet I now know it was the best. I had lost my home, my car, the church I was pastoring was shut down and the belongings that we did have in storage were damaged due to a broken pipe in the storage facility. I had been out of work for about a year and a half and I was back home living with one I hated, my mother. I had to move my daughter and I back into the room that I grew up in. When I went back into this room the nightmares of my childhood began to play before me like a movie. All of those old feelings of abandonment and rejection that I thought I had escaped from my moving out began to flood my memory. The verbal abuse that I had once experienced living with my Mother as a child began again. That spirit was back with a vengenance to let me know it still hated, me and wanted to kill me. Believe me there were many days will being back here that it felt like I wanted to die. I knew I had screwed up bad and was wondering if God would help me. I was a preacher of the gospel, speaking hope, and encouraging and exhorting others but could not find it in myself to encourage myself in the Lord. I had been on the verge of a nervous breakdown so many times, and probably did have one. I began to attend a ministry that dealt with spiritual warfare and was a very good teach ministry. When I got there I looked like I was ship wrecked. I did not even have anymore church clothes, but I had one white t-shirt and one pair of jeans that I kept clean and wore them until could get more. I began to get my strength back and I was learning how to fight. One day the leader of the ministry approached me and asked me to help open and mange their first business venture, a café. I was honored and nervous at the same time but I needed a job so I agreed. I jumped in with great zeal but had no idea of what all this would entail. I did not count the cost and had no idea all that God was going to show me in experience. I began once again to seek this leader's approval and love, hence erected another altar in my life that God would bring crashing down. I no longer believed in myself or in the power God for that matter. I had basically come to the end of myself. Why do I say that, because I always felt that if I did what someone wanted me to do I woule get in return the love and acceptance I was so depserately searching for. The fact of the matter is that we as believers erect altars to look up to or aspire to because we somehow lead ourselves to believe that they are going to be able to meet the innermost need that we crave after, to be loved, to be accpeted abd validated. Not looking for the healing of peace, which up until I had never heard of and did not even know that was what I needed. We began to cross lines and bounderies that would end up being very detrimental to our ministerial and professional relationship. But while I was working in the café, God did something for me. I found a book by the late Dr. Leon Sullivan, whom we refer to as the, "Lion in Zion" here in Philadelphia. The title of the book was, "Build Brother Build". One day something powerful lept off the page at me and if said, "If nobody else believes in you,

71

you believe in yourself". That was my wake call. I began to cry as I just said to myself, " I believe, I believe".

During this time my daughter, our neighborhood grandmother and myself had become avid fans of the TV show American Idol. We were rooting for Fantasia, she just had to win. And to my surprise the song that she sang for the finale was the cincher for me, the title of the song was, "I Believe". It wasa like God himself said let me bring this home for my Babygirl. When she sang that song on that she won she herself with new revelation, like yes now I am going to invest in myself too. That was such a defining moment in my life and I made sure as soon as the CD went on sale I purchased it to continually remind myself of the belief in what God had placed on the inside of me. Now I don't allow others to define my success because what you deem as successful many not be what I feel is successful. I would never impose that on anyone but I had allowed so many to impose their beliefs of success on me instead of hearing what God said about me and my success in Him. The word of God says in Jeremiah 29:11,

For I know the thoughts that I think toward you, saith the Lord, thoughts of peace, and not evil, to give you and expected end".

From that we understand that God wants us to be successful but in our own right, in the path He designed for each of us. How we get there is a journey but when we take our eyes off of other people's journey and concentrate on our own we will be so much better for it.

One day about a month ago I was waiting on the bus to go to work and someone rode by in their car playing a song I had not heard in a while. The name of the song is "I Wish" by R. Kelly. Whenever I hear this song I think of my grandmother, how I wish I could hold her, how I wish I could talk to her because so many things have happened in my life that I have seemed to be so unprepared for and man do I wish she was here. I stood at the bus stop crying big crocodile tears but I hurried myself to wipe my face. Now there are two reasons for that, one because I had on my make-up and I was looking too gorgeous this morning and two, what would people think? Hmmm, there I go worrying about people. This day I decided to forget all about them and cry. I had a right to cry I missed my mother/grandmother. So I cried, even on the trolley I cried and it felt so good to release it and not hold on to it. I cried until I for off at my stop about five blocks later. As I was walking up to my job God then said, "Now invite the healing of peace to come in". So I said, "Healing of peace, God I don't understand". You see I had invited people (men/women), places (church, religious systems and doctrine), and things (alcohol, sex and even food). By now I had gained sixty pounds of, "I'm depressed so I'll eat pounds) since I lost my mother/ grandmother but not the peace of God. He then said to me, "this is what Styllwater's is about, the waters represent me leading you in to this peace where there is healing". "This is why I birthed Styllwater's though you it just took this long to get to it. While many come for different reasons the underlying one is they come seeking the same peace for their own souls. That peace is the thing you have longed for, you have journeyed after it unknowingly and you are now about to bring them to a place where it can be invited in. You are just like them trying to work out your own soul's salvation (peace) just as they are".

Chapter 5

How Did I Get Here

You know we all have defining moments in our lives that let us know something is a stronghold in our life. It leads us into further investigation or at least it should. For me it came in my early twenties, there was a class being taught and members of the class were recovering addicts but then other people started to attend the class because the teaching of the Word was so good and they were able to apply it to your everyday life. Then one day I was at the teacher's house and stumbled onto an addict's bible. As I was reading the Bible I began to study the characteristics of and addict and what the road to deliverance entailed. While I was reading I discovered something, I was

addicted to sex.

It's out there now. I used sex, and masturbation as a stress reliever to escape from the pain of life just as an addict uses drugs, alcohol, and shopping or even food. Again it all starts in the mind and the imagination of the mind. And in many areas of my life as I look even now some of my addictions are more progressive than others. Because since I no longer have sex, I eat comfort foods to deal and find myself hiding behind that "I deserve this since I don't do this, this and that". Can we be real and admit we have all been guilty of this in one form or another. But the one thing I was forced to do at this time once I began to study the addiction battle was to go back to the root. This meant I had to revisit some painful places in my life and no one likes to do that. We do not like to do that because it requires us to look at ourselves. We can no longer play the blame game. It requires us to take ownership of our part in the matter and to examine why we do what we do. No one wants to readily admit to his or her faults because then you have the job of putting in place a plan of action to correct that behavior. Am I saying you leave God or the Holy Spirit out, no but God brings it to the light to let you know that it is now to time to deal with this thing that is in essence self-destructive and will cause you more harm than good.

Ever wake up and wonder like the song Deborah Cox sings, "How Did You Get Here"? That is the question I had to begin to ask myself because this addiction lead me to places I would love to say I would never go.

You know as I study the book of Judges and the life of Samson I learned some very important life lessons. Never lay your head down in the wrong lap. We can have a legitimate need in our lives but like Samson we can have that need met in an illegitimate way. The need to be loved and comforted is not a wrong thing but the way I set out to have those needs met was not always good. Samson's mother and Father were given specific instructions on how to raise him and they armed Samson with this information as well. Like us today we are raised with specific morals and the word of God but at some point we decide that we know what is best for us, we know better than God. I mean that He just does not wasn't us to have any fun and that is why He has all these rules for us to live by right? Absolutely not but at some point in our lives when we think we handle it we attempt to take the reigns of our lives and live on what we call on our own times not understanding the repercussions of our actions and what our disobedience will lead to. We take lightly the fact that whatever we are doing we are sowing seeds and they can be seeds of righteousness or seeds of unrighteousness but no matter what we are sowing. What then grows from those crops we have not idea but they can reek all kinds of havoc in your life and your bloodline.

Sometimes we eat things today that lead us to develop different appetites for tomorrow, good or not so well. Well I began to eat some things that were not too good for me and they were producing the wrong effect, things such: as self-pity, self-loathing, self-hatred, bitterness, resentment, grief, depression and despair. I was now attending the woe is me school and boy was I a good student. The thing about this school is no one in the class will admit or even challenge what the teacher (devil) is teaching because they love being there, it brings the very attention they desire which could be misunderstood as a good thing it was not a Godly thing. Because of this we make peopled co-dependent because they feed something in our own insecurities and inadequacies. We help them stay there because if they ever get out who will we now enlist to make us look like the victor we think we are instead of the victim we really are. We need to be honest and say we really need the help as much as they do too. Many times we believe when we go through the people we think are helping us need us more than we really think we need them but they may never let you know it. Moreover, the sad thing is they try to do the "remember when" thing on you when you start to gain the strength to begin to stand on your own again.

Please remember this, the way you meet someone or the condition you meet him or her in does not define them. Circumstances and situations are temporary they change just like the wind, just ask Job. You know most addicts were either introduced to or were curious about whatever they somehow became addicted to and it goes from there. I was introduced to sex at a very innocent age of four by my mother's boyfriend. I began to have sex on my own at five at my day-care in the teacher's bathroom/lounge with another of my classmates. When I was nine I was having intercourse with a fourteen-year-old boy could not even explain to me what the foamy stuff was. When I was fifteen I was kidnapped and raped. So from the door I never had a healthy outlook on sex. It began in a warped state and remained that way for some time. In between all of these events I was still going to church every Sunday and like the great Marvin Gaye always reiterated I still loved Jesus.

I firmly believe that I am not married to this day because of all of these issues and others surrounding my sexuality. God wants us to be totally delivered, healed and whole. That is what it means when the Bible says in **3 John 2:1 NKJV**,

"Beloved, I pray that you may prosper in all things and be in health, just as your soul prospers".

But if something is broken it cannot prosper properly. There will always be some part of the machine that does not operate at its fullest potential until it has been completely overhauled and repaired, made whole. I have been in the garage called Adullam for some time. You know I thought many issues that I dealt with in my life were because God was punishing me. Example, I thought if I sinned I lost my car. Never mind the fact that I did not keep up with the payments, if I had never sinned I would still have my car. Makes no sense at all right? But somewhere my train of thought was warped. It really led back to lack of self-control and discipline, which led to excessive behaviour, which then leads to sin. Anything in excess is a sin. Shopping, eating, drinking eating, etc. Boy that's deep. You see I will acknowledge that I was introduced to sex wrong but once I came into the saving knowledge of Jesus Christ and matured in the word of God those old things were supposed to pass away and all things were supposed to be made new. But I took old stuff into a new place. These old things complicated this wonderful new place. The Apostle Paul wrote it so eloquently about a runner and how he should run a race. Many times in the race of life there are: hurdle, obstacles, speed bumps, and even potholes and craters. How we navigate through these areas determine how well we run the race. When a runner approaches the starting block he/she is scantily clothed because they need as less as possible to pick up and maintain speed and they do not need anything weighing them down.

I Corinthian 9:24-27

Amplified Bible, Classic Edition

24 Do you not know that in a race all the runners compete, but [only] one receives the prize? So run [your race] that you may lay hold [of the prize] and make it yours.

25 Now every athlete who goes into training conducts himself temperately and restricts himself in all things. They do it to win a wreath that will soon wither, but we [do it to receive a crown of eternal blessedness] that cannot wither.

26 Therefore I do not run uncertainly (without definite aim). I do not box like one beating the air and striking without an adversary.

27 But [like a boxer] I buffet my body [handle it roughly, discipline it by hardships] and subdue it, for fear that after proclaiming to others the Gospel and things pertaining to it, I myself should become unfit [not stand the test, be unapproved and rejected as a counterfeit].

In our lives when we don't address behaviour that is detrimental to our well being, we begin to see a pattern developing. A pattern that will lead us to a path of sure destruction if we do not take head to the warning signs and make the necessary adjustments. Just as Samson did not take heed I did not always take head to the warning signs. To be honest I did not want to because I had a legitimate need that God took too long to address so I decided to take it upon myself because I needed to feel the way my "Delilah's" made me feel: My "Delilah's" made me feel loved, accepted and understood. They helped me to escape the pain of grief, abandonment, and rejection. I did not care that this was a temporary fix for issues that I should have been seeking a permanent one for. I just like the way my "Delilah's" made me feel no matter what the expense. I will say it again it was something beautiful and enticing that filled a legitimate need in the wrong way.

I use the term "Delilah's" loosely because we all have something that we lean on or look to make us feel better that is not good for us. That "lap" was not an ordained rest stop for us because of that the end result did not yield us the results we were expecting. We really get more than we bargained for when we do that. I did not always use self-control and as we will discuss in the next chapter how that lead to me to "laps" I never even imagined I would sink to but I did. It was in the midst of those places I learned some very hard truths about God, my character and most of all myself.

Chapter 6

Never Say Never

Because I could not be patient and allow God to heal me and the holes in my heart I continued on my self-destructive path. That led me to the place I never envisioned that I would be in is that I found myself in; and that was in an lesbian relationship with a married woman. How did I get here? By never dealing with and addressing all the signs along the road that leads to this point. By not subduing and taking dominion over my flesh and make it come subject to the Holy Spirit on the inside of me. By not taking head to the signs of rebellion in the other areas of my life that seemed to cross over more and more into other areas until there were no longer any boundaries. It was just like since things are not coming the way I want them to I will settle for this. So I settled. I began to believe the lie and the myth that since my mother never loved me, my grandmother had left me and my baby daddy had walked out on me, it was only fair that someone loved me and what did it matter if it was a woman. No matter that she was married and had children. This manifestion happened immediately following my initial trial sermon. I did not pay attention to the fact that in the infancy of my ministry that the enemy was seeking to destroy me from the womb just as he had sought to do in the natural.

I was always affectionate and needy because my mother was never affectionate towards me and neither was my grandmother to tell the truth. I remember telling my grandmother one day that she never told me she loved me. She thought because she showed me and that I should have known. After I made that revelation known I must say she made more of an effort to day it But once she died the spirit of rejection that had lurked around me for so long was looking for an entry way and had found room. I believed that there was no one left on this earth that loved me. I was so convinced that my mother hated me that I even asked her one day why she didn't abort me. You must understand that I had endured so much hurt and pain looking in the eyes of a woman that never seemed to love or accept me which drove me into the arms of many people and the unlitmate a woman. I was not seeking a lesbian relationship, I was seeking a motherly relationship but you know how it is you give me what I need and I'll give you what you need. The same way it in a male/female relationship. Still twisted and perverted. Many times church women have preyed on other women who are only looking for a natural need and make it an ungodly need. A legitimate need met in and illegitimate way. It is unnatural for you to prostitute that person in their weak moment for your gratification. I am not playing the victim I am just sharing to enlighten and educate God's people how spirit's manifest and what their root causes are.

I was becoming a castaway, I was preaching to others but yet moving further and further away from what I was preaching and teaching. I was in such a war withing myself. I kept seeing my grandmother's face and feeling I had disappointed her. I kept hearing her say,

"I did not raise you like this". But I kept saying, "But you left me here all alone". "I have nothing and no one"

And even in those moments I knew I did not have this woman because she was married. In this process I tried to get out of this relationship at least 50 times. I kept going over and over it in my head. I kept thinking about the ramifications in the spirit for our children. I wanted to break so many curses and not have them pass down to my daughter yet here I ws bringing something new into the mix. This woman's children did not deserve this and not to mention her husband. He loved me and took me as his sister. He welcomed me into his home. We even lived there for sometime while my daughter and I were in transition. And yes we even slept together under their roof. My mind was so twisted to the point where I began to justify this thing and say, "Well she was unhappy, he didn't love her right and that she deserved to be happy". I was just happy that I had somebody and they loved me back. Atleast that is what the enemy lead me to believe. It was an legitimate need met in an illegitimate way. I began to buy into the lie that she was mine and it was ok as long as we had each other, who cared what the world had to say about it.

It took me years to walk through the deliverance process of this stronghold because every time I almost made to the door something pulled me back. The attention, the affection, and rejection in some other areas of my life just seemed to facilitate this relationship. I could not let go and it really got to a very dangerous place when I did not even want to hear God or care about the consequences of this grievious relationship. I say grievous, because it grieved my spirit as well as the Holy Spirit. We started dating as a couple in the red light district, going to parties with friends who were in the same circle but never came out completely and allowed our relationship to be public knowledge. My partner was afraid of what would happen because of the hate crimes that homosexuals were often the victims of so she would not be openly affectionate in public, which drove me crazy. I felt she was just playing a power game with the relationship to get what she wanted when it was good for her. She tortured me when she was angry and was very affectionate with her husband in front of me when she wanted to teach me a lesson but did not want me to have any friends. The relationship was very possessive but eventually I got tired of seeing her husband take her to bed and not being able to do anything about it. Because the bottom line of it all was: one he was her husband and two this was a unnatural affair that God was not going to bless and that I had better get out of it before I got to the place of no return. I was pretty close as it was and I knew that I had to make some changes fast. But she kept coming to me complaining about how unhappy she was, how he raped her in bed, how he did not provide romance in the relationship. Then I would run to her rescue and try to make everything alright and try to woo her back to me and make her believe that I was so much better for her and would love her so much more than her husband would.

We were both at a new church and were trying to start all over again. I had told my new Pastor the events of the previous church but did not tell him that the woman was there with me also. This is what I learned was calculated truth, not telling all of the truth and until you do that you can never be completely free, healed or delivered. So once again I was in the way of my deliverance that I claimed I wanted so badly. I do believe I wanted it but I wanted it on my own terms. I wanted to keep her in my life, somehow in my mind I believed we could still be friends and act like nothing had ever happened; which was not at all possible at this time.

I feel the need to stop here and say something for the brothers. It is not unnatural for them to seek out affirmation and acceptance from male role models or leaders either. Because if we think about it, in some way we all find ourselves looking for something that is missing in our lives. Just like in our natural bodies when we are not getting enough protein or vitamins we will find ourselves craving for food that has those ingredients that we are missing. Predators prey on others because they are hungry or have a need. But the predators are not going after the food source in the spirit. So it becomes a vicious cycle and the void never gets filled. Can we just be real admitting we all want to be loved and accepted and we are not that holy and spiritual that these issues do not touch us? If they did not and were not intended to touch us we would not have the examples in the Bible such as the woman at the well. God knew He had a whole lot of daughters and sons that were going to come after her that were going to need to meet the Man that would stop them from seeking water from any other well. But just like the woman at the well we try to play word games with the Holy Spirit or as one of my mentors call it and I love this expression, "calculated truth" games to side step the issue. Some of us want to come by night like Nicodemus, but however you come to get your drink just make sure you come.

SIDEBAR

The house next to my Mother is a speakeasy. Something like a ghetto juke joint. When the red light is on you can get whatever you need but if it is off don't ring the bell. What I love about Jesus is that His light is always on.

I am going to go back to something I discussed earlier in the chapter. It was regarding Samson and him laying his head on Delilah's lap. I have been traveling a lot on the Greyhound bus lately and there is one thing that stays consistent, they have scheduled rest stops. They know at some point the drivers are going to need a break, and that the passengers will need to stretch their legs use the facilities. The bus company anticipates this, but if the stop is not on the schedule it is unauthorized and the driver will have to answer for it to a higher authority. Not just for his bus but for the safety of the passengers that are in his hands. So I say all of that to say this, there are authorized stops in our journey that God has ordained for us because He knows we get tired, and need to be refreshed and renewed.

But there are also some stops that God does not authorize when we feel in our own flesh that we are not able to go on. During those times we usually are feeling that way because we have not been in our Word, been in God's presence, or fasting like we should. So we become weak and malnourished because our diet has changed and head towards the first mirage that the enemy shows us. A mirage is something that looks like it is there but really is not there. Delilah was not there for Samson she just looked like she was there for him but she was really there as a spy to find out the secret to his strength. She was paid to do this because the Philistines could not attack Israel as long as Samson had his strength. They knew they could get to Israel if they got to Samson. So each Philistine lord paid

Delilah 1,100 shekels, which amounted to 5,500 shekels. In American money that is $46,307.80. Samson was worth that much to move out of the way to the Philistine lords. How much are you worth to the enemy to have moved out of the way?

Samson's needs were a mirage used by the enemy to move him out of position. The need was legitimate but where he lay his head was a mirage, it was not real or Delilah would not have been able to betray him. She may have loved him but that the plots and schemes of the enemy perverted the love. Samson was deceived by the mirage because he wanted his needs met even if it was illegitimately done.

The definition of a mirage is:

an optical effect that is sometimes see at sea, in the desert, or over a hot pavement, that may have the appearance of a pool of water or a mirror in which distant objects are seen inverted, and that is caused by the bending or reflection of rays of light by a layer of heated air varying density. 2. Something illusory and unattainable like a mirage desert experience, wilderness, and dry place.

Have you ever noticed in these valleys or low place experiences that instead of dealing with the reality of what we are the enemy shows us something that is not and makes you believe there is a possibility that it could be? For example, instead of allowing your process on the potter's wheel to keep spinning until the image that God is trying to bring forth is formed, the enemy tempts us with the thoughts of how we can get off early. After all, all of the things we are experiencing are not our fault and we deserve some happiness in our lives. The truth of the matter is that happiness is overrated and temporal but joy is everlasting. We just do not remember these important nuggets in our valley places because in those times and I must admit we are led more and more by our emotions then by the spirit of the Living God. Even Jesus was led into the wilderness and tempted. So why do we think we will not be tempted? But in His greatest temptations Jesus gave the enemy the Word. We do not always revert back to that when the enemy comes to us with his barrage of thoughts and accusations about what God is doing or not doing on our behalf. We forget that God's word says that He knows the plans that He has for us and they are not to harm us but to bring us to an expected end. We just do not know what the expected end entails and it sees to take so long that we often times decide we need to help God out like Sarah. We end up doing more harm than good and find ourselves like the children of Israel having to wander in the wilderness for however many years until we allow patience to have her perfect work. I found a lot about myself in this wilderness place. I was selfish, self-centred and only cared about what would make me feel better, my needs being met. I had abandoned all morals and became such a hypocrite. I got angry when people talked about me in my situation. I tried to hide behind the persecution for righteousness thing but I was so far from that. One thing in specific God began to deal with me about is what do you do when people tell the truth about you? Nobody really wants believe that they have sunk to this place but it is the truth. You are then forced to look at the reality of you in the mirror and have to say I do not like what I see. So I tried to do something about it but was not completely willing to do all that I should have done.

One day I went to see the movie Titanic and while watching the movie I saw something that reminded me so much of myself. One of the characters Rose had the opportunity to get off of the boat would not leave without Jack. Although we may have loved the character Jack, Rose knew that she had already made a commitment to another man. While the boat was lowering Rose jumped back onto a sinking Titanic because she could not see herself going on without Jack. I myself was Rose on a sinking ship. I had the opportunity many times to get off but I kept fumbling my deliverance process many times because I could not see myself going on without this woman. What was it about her? It was like I was under a spell or something every time I wanted to set away I somehow could not bring myself to do it. I went into counselling and the minister told me to repeat something three times and then it would break. Nothing happened and I went out expecting something to be different. And I think the thing that devastated me the most is that the minister called and told my pastor about my transgression before I did and it began to spread like wildfire. She then blamed me for my pastor no longer associating with her because she appeared guilty by association, which was a crock of crap. This sent me spiralling even the more into oblivion because I felt there was no place safe for me to get help. So life in my church became a witch-hunt, scandal ridden and just very stressful. People even began to mistreat my 2-year old daughter because of my indiscretion. In the midst of this the woman's husband began to beat her and it killed me to watch her go through this. The men and pastor of the church felt it was justified and basically closed their eyes to this. Her children were very confused, and so were those who looked to me as a minister who had fallen away from grace. When I took this fall this was the unspeakable in my mind I wondered many times how I could ever recover from this one. Yet in the midst of this I knew God would use it for His glory. But at this time His glory was not a consoling thought. My character and integrity in ministry were shot before I even got the chance to begin. I was living in between two worlds. I even began to visit the red light district where our relationship would be accepted and still went to church on Sunday. I began to buy into the lie that God must had intended for me to be like this, why else would I have these feelings and urges. I wanted to marry this woman, buy a house and raise our children together. I was pretty far gone into this thing. But then something happened, her husband wanted to fight for his marriage so I was in competition with him. I began to try to out buy him in every way. Flowers, candy, dinner and movies, you name it I did it. Now you know I really lost my mind. The Holy Spirit brought back to my remembrance how David stole Uriah's wife and could have anyone else in the kingdom but chose his wife. Her husband was trying to find his way in Christ and here I was a minister in the church contending with him for his lamb. Even as I read while I write I am in disbelief of how far sin had taken me. I really believe I was extremely close to where the Apostle Paul in the book of Romans chapter one speaks about being turned over to their own lust and then eventually a reprobate mind. Somehow even knowing this I still tried to precede and do things my own way. I had long lost my sense of direction and yet even in this Christ was still my compass. I was just refusing to yield to the direction He was trying to steer me in. So I fully understand when Hezekiah Walker's choir sings, "Oh Lord I've sinned but I still hear you calling my name". Greatness and destiny were still calling me even in this state, which was far beyond my belief. I had the most anointed dreams in this period of my life much like Jacob when he slept and saw the angels ascending and descending. I would see angels in my dreams that just repeating, "Blessings, blessings, blessings". In my mind I was like who me, they must be in the wrong place. But I really did know if was the Lord. By this time in my life I had been through so many things. My apartment had been robbed twice, my car was stolen and finances were in extreme lack. As was the woman I was involved with. I was trying hard to raise my beautiful daughter without the help of her father and no support from my own family. So here you had two crutches trying to hold each other up. Hard times make strange bedfellows. Don't know who said it but I do know it to be true. When I finally allowed the Lord to show me myself, it really blew my mind. My feelings were hurt because no one likes to see how messed up and ugly they truly are. But the revelation God gave me one weekend while in Pittsburgh was that I was a love junkie looking for another high.

Once that high was over I would seek another. No matter how much negative or positive attention it caused; I just wanted the high, the attention, I wanted my needs met by any means necessary. This is a very dangerous place because if you are not careful you will find yourself concocting things to draw attention to you in some form or another. Whether the relationship is real or imaginary. Making problems appear bigger than they are so that you I will appear to need so much help and once people do come to rescue me I become labelled as the boy /girl who cried wolf. A junkie meaning taking something that is no good for you and will not last and trying to make it fix what the real circumstances are. It is an escape from reality, living in a false world. So that still means that the imagination in the mind still needs to be cast down so that God can come and do the total healing and restoration work. It's like a computer once it crashes it needs to be rebooted. My spirit, soul and mind needed a reboot.

Chapter 7

Break Through

Experience

One day I cried out to God and really meant it and He met me where I was. But that was not until I began to confess my truth about myself. The ugly truth, not the altered version I had rehearsed to myself over and over to justify my broken life. Then it was like every day I found myself getting stronger and stronger and able to deny myself what my flesh seemed to crave, connection and acceptance no matter what. How did I get out of a lesbian relationship, I finally ran out like a dog scalded with hot water. I kept crying out to God on my face with one of my sister's in Christ and like I said earlier I really meant it. I wanted my total and complete deliverance from a spirit that was trying to over take me in every area of my life. When you look at the story of Samson the spirit of "Delilah" came to completely destroy him because if there was no one at the gate the enemy could rampage the Children of Israel. I came to an awakening that I was needed at my gate and if I was not in place the enemy could have a field day with those whom I was called to guard in the spirit. This was all about my purpose, the cause for which I was born. I was not haphazardly put into my Mother's womb, it was by divine design because there was a cause, a purpose for me that only I could fulfil because what was needed was placed on the inside of me by God. Remember Ephesians 4:1 says, "that before the foundations of the world God chose us to be in Him. I was already in Him and will remain but the next part of the verse says He called us to be holy. He called us to be holy, not perfect but holy. It's true when the Bible says that some things only come by prayer and fasting and this spirit is one of them and I needed to abstain from it and every evil that would lead you back to this pit. Did I ever look back, yes. Did I ever go back, yes. Because it had become a part of my nature and I had to make a daily choice to die to it every day if I really meant what I said to God and that was I wanted to get out. I had to aggressively fight in the spirit realm for my femininity because I was called to birth life and enemy was trying to pervert my God ordained purpose in life. We as women are called to carry life and men are called to give life. If you change roles you are not able to produce that you were designed to produce. I had to fight to be the Mother I was called to be and impart natural truths to my daughter on what a woman is supposed to be. If I had stayed in this lifestyle it was not only going to affect my generation but the one coming behind me and God only knows how many more until someone broke the curse. I had to fight because God said that I was more than a conqueror and that I had already won the battle against this spirit I just had to walk it out. I had to fight because society and even the church world said I could not have this kind of relationship, get delivered, set free and stay free.

The Bible says in ***Revelations 12:11 AMP***

"And they overcame him by the blood of the lamb and the words of our testimony".

I have overcome because of the blood of the lambs and these words of my testimony. I have a testimony of what my Daddy can do and He said that now is the time for me to step forward and tell about what only He can do, the miraculous. What you say is impossible God says with Him is possible. God is no respecter of persons what He has done for me He can do for you too. I still have to stay on my face daily to be able to withstand my test and trials because the enemy always comes to see if you are dead in your flesh. I did not get through because God gave me a man, but I got through it because God delivered me. I give all glory and honor to Him. Do people still label me, yes but I am healed. Do they want to always remember my past, yes but I am healed. Do I fight not to go back to my past, yes but I am healed. Since it was God that did the healing, my only job is to walk out my healing.

My relationship with my Mother is being healed, my relationship with food, finances, self- worth and self-esteem are being healed.

Paul said it best in *Philippians 3:13-14 KJV*

"Brethren I count not myself to have apprehended but this one thing I do, forgetting those things which are behind and reaching forth unto those things which are before, I press toward the mark for the prize of the high calling of God in Christ Jesus"

I am not perfect but I am being perfected because of the Christ in me the perfected One.

About the Author

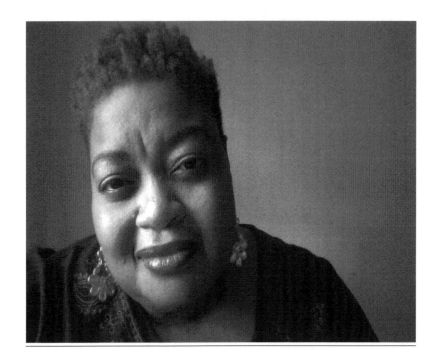

Ramona M. Gaines is the founder and CEO of Styllwaters' Café Inc. and Styllwaters' Ministries a non-profit-organization that provides a venue for Christian artist to perform and network. The Styllwaters' Story, Ramona's first book is the inspirational story of life, and passion that lead her to establish the Styllwaters' Café.

A seasoned entrepreneur, Gaines operates Parent Kids Network, which specializes in restoring and transforming the lives of parents and children by instilling family values and offering structural guidance that not only builds strong families but strong communities.

As the visionary of Movement is Medicine, Gaines not only seeks to inspire others but create a movement through a compilation of stories about how a commitment to move daily can become the medicine to overcome spiritual, physical, mental and emotional challenges. The powerful series includes Movement Is Medicine: Volume I, Women Determined to Rise: Volume II and Men Determined to Break Free: Volume III parallels Chicken Soup for the Soul as it takes readers on a journey of spiritual, physical and emotional transformation.

A native of Philadelphia, Pennsylvania, Gaines

attended Millersville University where she studied Radio and Television Broadcasting. Gaines also attended Manna Bible School, Present Truth Ministries School of Ministry and she is certified Trauma Specialist at The Institute of Family Professionals at Lakeside Education Network.

Gaines is the parent of one daughter, Ellana Monae' and the proud of Auntie of over 10 nieces and nephews.

Made in the USA
Middletown, DE
30 October 2017